THE MEDITERRANEAN DIET COOKBOOK

50 Best Recipes to Introduce Yourself to the Mediterranean Alimentation and Ingredients

Healthy & Lovely

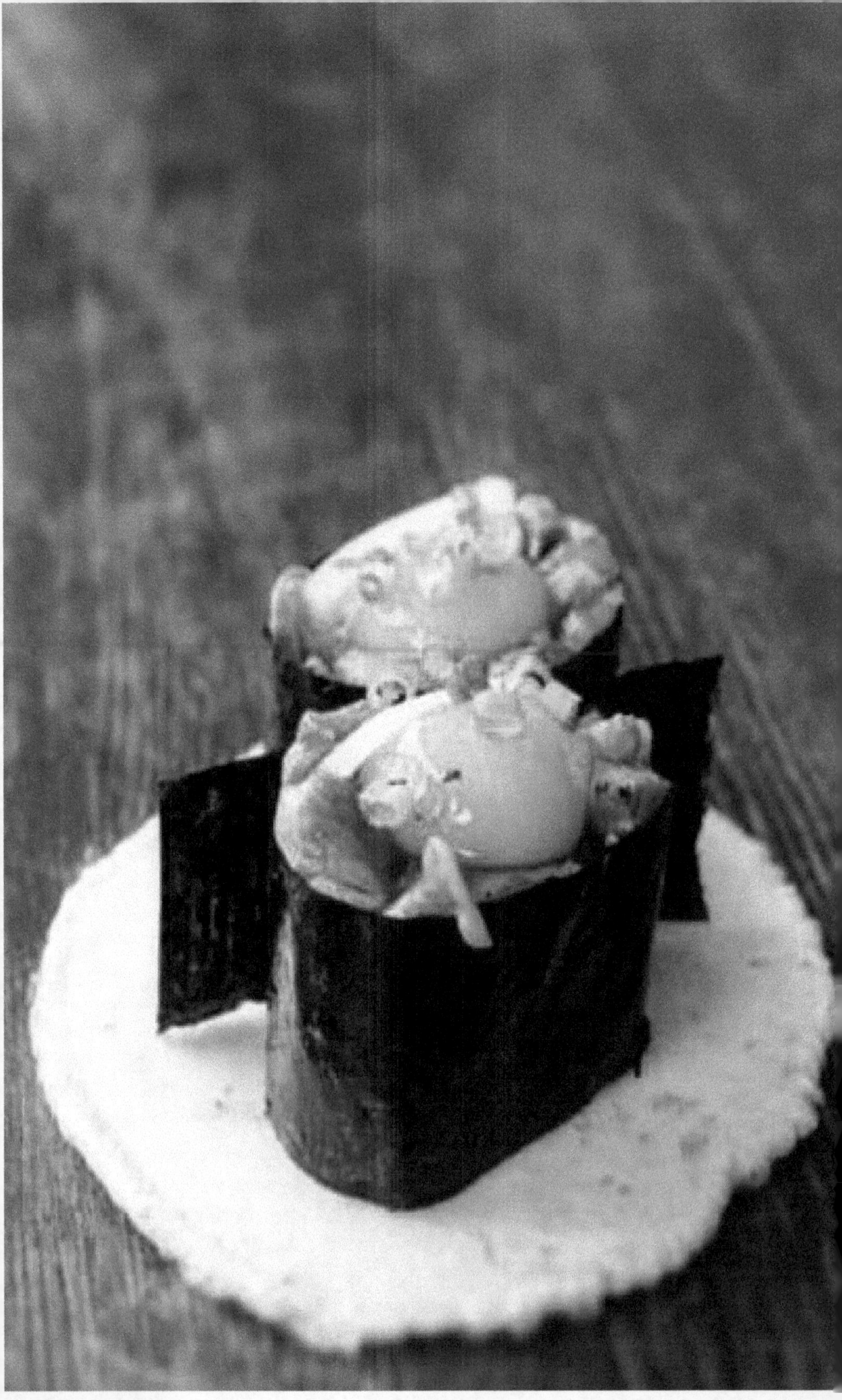

inattention, use, or misuse of the information in question by the reader will render any resulting actions solely under their purview. There are no scenarios in which the publisher or the original author of this work can be in any fashion deemed liable for any hardship or damages that may befall them after undertaking information described herein.

Additionally, the information in the following pages is intended only for informational purposes and should thus be thought of as universal. As befitting its nature, it is presented without assurance regarding its prolonged validity or interim quality. Trademarks that are mentioned are done without written consent and can in no way be considered an endorsement from the trademark holder.

Table of Contents

INTRODUCTION

Mediterranean Diet

A Mediterranean diet incorporates the traditional healthy living habits of people from countries bordering the Mediterranean Sea, including France, Greece, Italy, and Spain. A traditional diet from the Mediterranean region includes a generous portion of fresh produce, whole grains, and legumes, as well as some healthful fats and fish. In general, it's high in vegetables, fruits, legumes, nuts, beans, cereals, grains, fish, and unsaturated fats such as olive oil. It usually includes a low intake of meat and dairy foods.

When you think about Mediterranean food, your mind may go to pizza and pasta from Italy or lamb chops from Greece, but these dishes don't fit into the healthy dietary plans advertised as "Mediterranean." That's how the inhabitants of Crete, Greece, and Southern Italy ate circa 1960, when their rates of chronic disease were among the lowest in the world and their life expectancy among the highest, despite having only limited medical services.

And the real Mediterranean diet is about more than just eating fresh, wholesome food. Daily physical activity and sharing meals with others are vital elements. Together, they can have a profound effect on your mood and mental health and help you foster a deep appreciation for the pleasures of eating healthy and delicious foods.

Of course, making changes to your diet is rarely easy, especially if you're trying to move away from the convenience of processed and takeout foods. But the Mediterranean diet can be an inexpensive as well as a satisfying and very healthy way to eat. Making the switch from pepperoni and pasta to fish and avocados may take some effort, but you could soon be on the path to a healthier and longer life.

If you have a chronic condition like heart disease or high blood pressure, your doctor may even have prescribed it to you. It is often promoted to decrease the risk of heart disease, depression, and dementia.

Research has consistently shown that the Mediterranean diet is effective in reducing the risk of cardiovascular diseases and overall mortality. [3, 4] A study of nearly 26,000 women found that those who followed this type of diet had 25 percent less risk of developing cardiovascular disease over the course of 12 years. [5] The study examined a range of underlying mechanisms that might account for this reduction, and found that changes in inflammation, blood sugar, and body mass index were the biggest drivers.

Tip for Making Your Diet More Mediterranean

You can make your diet more Mediterranean-style by:

- Including fish in your diet
- Choosing products made from vegetable and plant oils, such as olive oil
- Eating plenty of fruit and vegetables
- Eating plenty of starchy foods, such as bread and pasta
- Eating less meat
- Eating less dairy products
- Eating less packaged foods

Avoid the Following Foods If You Are on a Mediterranean Diet

- Foods with added sugars, such as pastries, sodas, and candies
- Refined grains such as white bread, white pasta, and pizza dough containing white flour
- Processed or packaged foods
- Refined oils, which include canola oil and soybean oil
- Deli meats, hot dogs, and other processed meats
- Dairy products

Benefits of Following a Mediterranean Diet

- Can help fight against cancer, diabetes, and cognitive decline
- Reduces the risk of Parkinson's disease
- Increases longevity
- Reduces the risk of Alzheimer's
- Protects against type 2 diabetes
- Prevents heart diseases and strokes
- Keeps you agile

Tips for a Quick Start to a Mediterranean Diet

The easiest way to make the change to a Mediterranean diet is to start with small steps.

You can do this by:

- Limit high-fat dairy by switching to skim or 1% milk.
- Eating more fruits and vegetables by enjoying salad as a starter or side dish, snacking on fruit, and adding veggies to other dishes.
- Choosing whole grains instead of refined breads, rice, and pasta.
- Sautéing food in olive oil instead of butter.
- Substituting fish for red meat at least twice per week.
- Prefer vegetables instead of meat.

1-Week Mediterranean Meal Plan

Monday

Breakfast

Greek yogurt with strawberries and oats

Lunch

Whole-grain sandwich with vegetables

Dinner

A tuna salad, dressed in olive oil, fruit for dessert

Tuesday

Breakfast

Oatmeal with raisins

Lunch

Leftover tuna salad from the night before

Dinner

Salad with tomatoes, olives, and feta cheese

Wednesday

Breakfast

Omelet with veggies, tomatoes and onions, a piece of fruit

Lunch

Whole-grain sandwich with cheese and fresh vegetables

Dinner

Mediterranean lasagna

Thursday

Breakfast

Yogurt with sliced fruits and nuts

Lunch

Leftover lasagna

Dinner

Broiled salmon, served with brown rice and vegetables

Friday

Breakfast

Eggs and vegetables fried in olive oil

Lunch

Greek yogurt with strawberries, oats, and nuts

Dinner

Grilled lamb with salad and baked potato

Saturday

Breakfast

Oatmeal with raisins, nuts, and an apple

Lunch

Whole-grain sandwich with vegetables

Dinner

Mediterranean pizza made with whole wheat, topped with cheese, vegetables, and olives

BREAKFAST

Raspberry Sauce & Vanilla Crepes

Servings: 4

Preparation Time: 15 minutes

Per Serving: Calories 425, Fat 34.1g; Total Carbs 20g; Protein 9.8g

Ingredients:

Crepes

- 1 tsp baking powder
- 1 cup milk
- 4 large eggs
- 1 cup flour
- ½ tsp salt
- 1 tbsp sugar
- 2 tbsps olive oil
- 1 tsp vanilla extract

Raspberries Sauce

- 2 tbsps sugar
- ½ cup water + 1 tbsp
- 3 cups fresh raspberries

- Juice of ½ lemon
- water
- ½ tsp cornstarch

Procedure:

1. In a bowl, mix the flour, salt, sugar, and baking powder with a whisk, and set aside.
2. In another bowl, whisk the milk, eggs, and vanilla extract together.
3. Pour the egg mixture into the flour mixture and continue whisking until smooth.
4. Preheat the griddle pan over medium heat and grease with olive oil.
5. Pour 1 soup spoonful of crepe batter into the griddle pan.
6. Cook on one side for 2 minutes, flip the crepe and cook the other side for 1 minute until brown and crispy.
7. Transfer the crepe to a plate and repeat the cooking process until the batter is exhausted.
8. Pour the raspberries and half cup of water into a saucepan, and bring the berries to boil over medium heat for about 8 minutes.
9. Lower the heat and simmer the berries for 5 minutes so that they are soft and exuding juice.

10. Pour in the sugar at this point, stir, and continue cooking for 5 minutes.
11. Next, stir in the lemon juice, and while they cook, mix the cornstarch with the remaining water; pour the mixture into the berries.
12. Stir and continue cooking the sauce to thicken to your desire. Turn off the heat and let it cool.
13. Finally, plate the crepes one on another and generously drizzle the raspberry sauce over them and serve.

Cheesy Spread Cinnamon Waffles

Servings: 12

Preparation Time: 25 minutes

Per Serving: Calories 495, Fat 48.5g; Total Carbs 16g; Protein 13g

Ingredients:

- 1 tsp baking powder
- 3 cups flour
- 16 oz mascarpone, at room temperature
- 14 large eggs
- 2 tsps cinnamon powder
- 6 tbsps brown sugar
- Cinnamon powder for garnishing
- 10 tbsps olive oil, melted
- 3 cups milk
- 1/2 tsp sugar

Procedure:

1. Whisk the olive oil, milk, and eggs in a medium bowl. Add the sugar and baking powder and mix.

2. Stir in the flour and combine until no lumps exist.
3. Spritz a waffle iron with cooking spray.
4. Ladle a ¼ cup of the batter into the waffle iron and cook until golden, about 10 minutes in total.
5. Repeat with the remaining batter.
6. Combine the mascarpone, cinnamon, and swerve with a hand mixer until smooth.
7. Cover and chill until ready to use.
8. Slice the waffles into quarters; apply the cheesy spread in between each of two waffles and snap.
9. Sprinkle with cinnamon powder and serve.

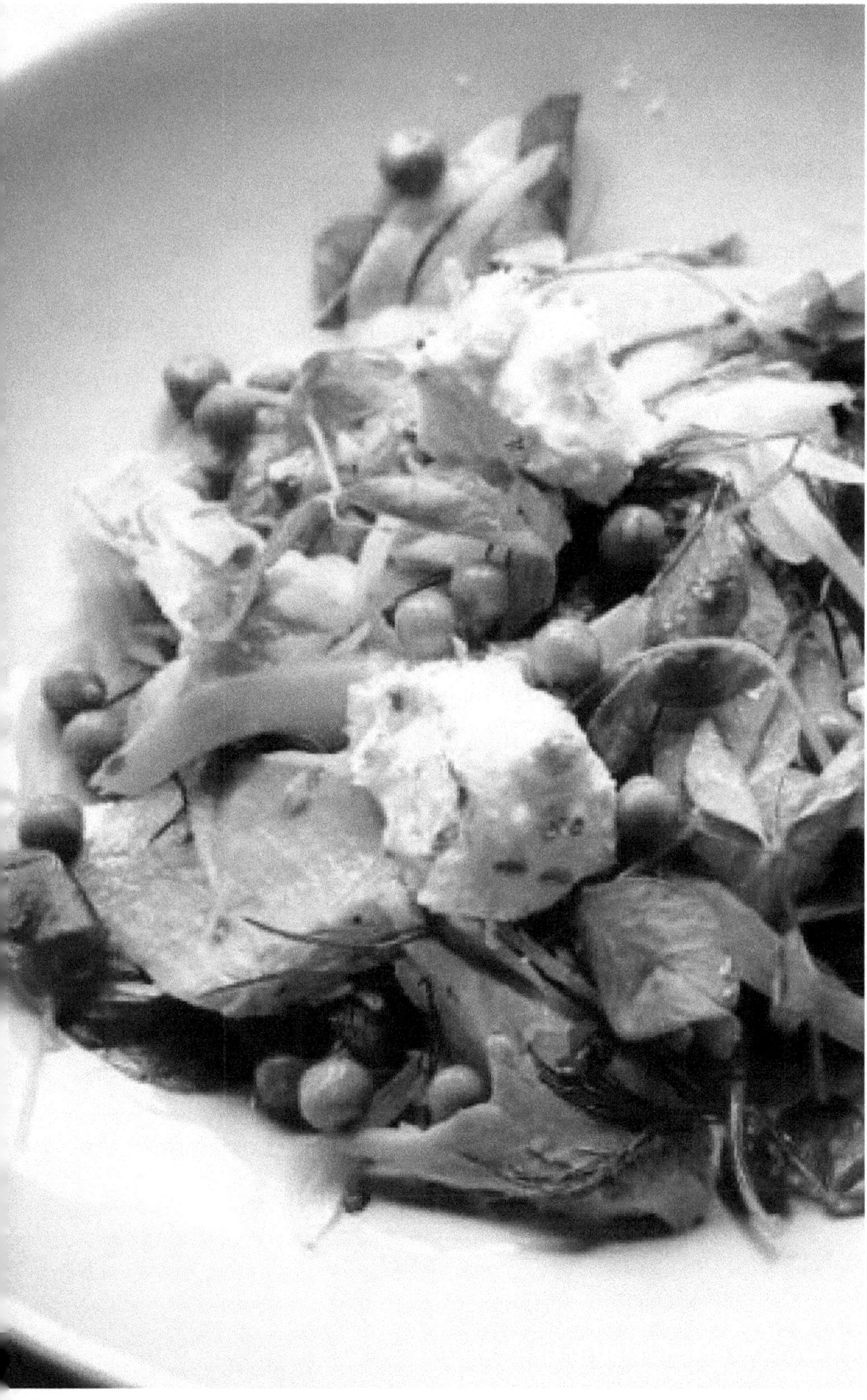

Rigatoni, Pea & Trout Morning Bowl

Servings: 8

Preparation Time: 15 minutes

Per Serving: Calories 350, Fat 6g; Total Carbs 27g; Protein 18g

Ingredients:

- 4 tbsps olive oil
- Salt to taste
- 2 cups green peas
- 32 oz rigatoni
- Zest and juice of 1 small lemon
- 6 oz smoked trout, fliked
- 12 Kalamata olives, pitted and sliced
- 6 tsps fresh dill, chopped

Procedure:

1. First, place a pot with salted water over medium heat and bring to a boil.
2. Add in the rigatoni and cook for 6 minutes.
3. Pour in the green peas and continue cooking until the pasta until is 'al dente', 3-4 more minutes.

4. Drain and transfer to a bowl.

5. Drizzle with olive oil and mix to coat.

6. Stir in smoked trout, Kalamata olive, lemon zest and juice.

7. Sprinkle with dill and serve.

Morning Egg Casserole

Servings: 4

Preparation Time: 40 minutes

Per Serving: Calories 68, fat 4.5, fiber 1, carbs 4.4, protein 3.4

Ingredients:

- ½ teaspoon salt
- 1 teaspoon paprika
- 1 tablespoon fresh cilantro, chopped
- 1 garlic clove, diced
- 1 chili pepper, chopped
- ½ red onion, diced
- 1 teaspoon canola oil
- 1 teaspoon butter, softened
- ¼ teaspoon chili flakes
- 2 eggs, beaten
- 1 red bell pepper, chopped

Procedure:

1. Brush the casserole mold with canola oil and pour beaten eggs inside.

2. After this, toss the butter in the skillet and melt it over medium heat.
3. Add chili pepper and red bell pepper.
4. After this, add red onion and cook the vegetables for 7-8 minutes over medium heat.
5. Stir them from time to time.
6. Transfer the vegetables in the casserole mold.
7. Add salt, paprika, cilantro, diced garlic, and chili flakes. Stir gently with the help of a spatula to get a homogenous mixture.
8. Bake the casserole for 20 minutes at 355F in the oven.
9. Then chill the meal well and cut into servings.
10. Transfer the casserole in the serving plates with the help of the spatula.

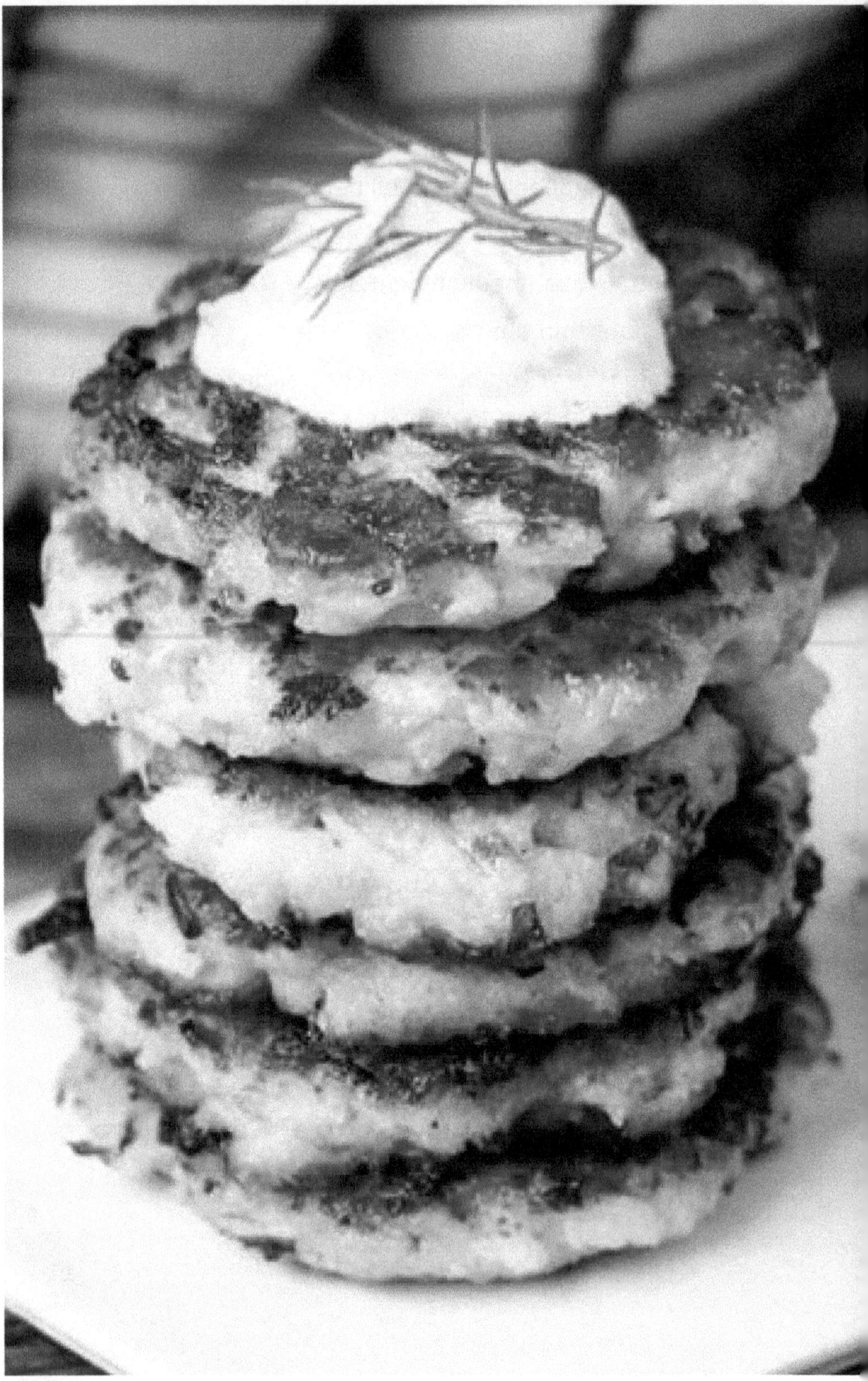

Cauliflower Fritters

Servings: 2

Preparation Time: 20 minutes

Per Serving: Calories 167, fat 12.3, fiber 1.5, carbs 6.7, protein 8.8

Ingredients:

- 1 oz Parmesan, grated
- ½ teaspoon ground black pepper
- 1 cup cauliflower, shredded
- 1 egg, beaten
- 1 tablespoon wheat flour, whole grain
- 1 tablespoon canola oil

Procedure:

1. In the mixing bowl, mix up together shredded cauliflower and egg.
2. Add wheat flour, grated Parmesan, and ground black pepper.
3. Stir the mixture with the help of the fork until it is homogenous and smooth.

4. Pour canola oil in the skillet and bring it to boil.
5. Make the fritters from the cauliflower mixture with the help of the fingertips or use a spoon and transfer in the hot oil.
6. Roast the fritters for 4 minutes from each side over medium-low heat.

Healthy Creamy Bulgur with Berries

Servings: 4

Preparation Time: 12 minutes

Per Serving: calories: 173 | fat: 1.6g | protein: 5.7g | carbs: 34.0g | fiber: 6.0g | sodium: 197mg

Ingredients:

- 2 teaspoons pure vanilla extract
- 1/2 teaspoon ground cinnamon
- 2 cups fresh berries of your choice
- 1 cup medium-grain bulgur wheat
- 2 cups water
- Pinch sea salt
- 1/2 cup unsweetened almond milk

Procedure:

1. First, put the bulgur in a medium saucepan with the water and sea salt, and bring to a boil.
2. Then cover, remove from heat, and let stand for 10 minutes until water is absorbed.

3. Now stir in the milk, vanilla, and cinnamon until fully incorporated.
4. Divide between 4 bowls and top with the fresh berries to serve.

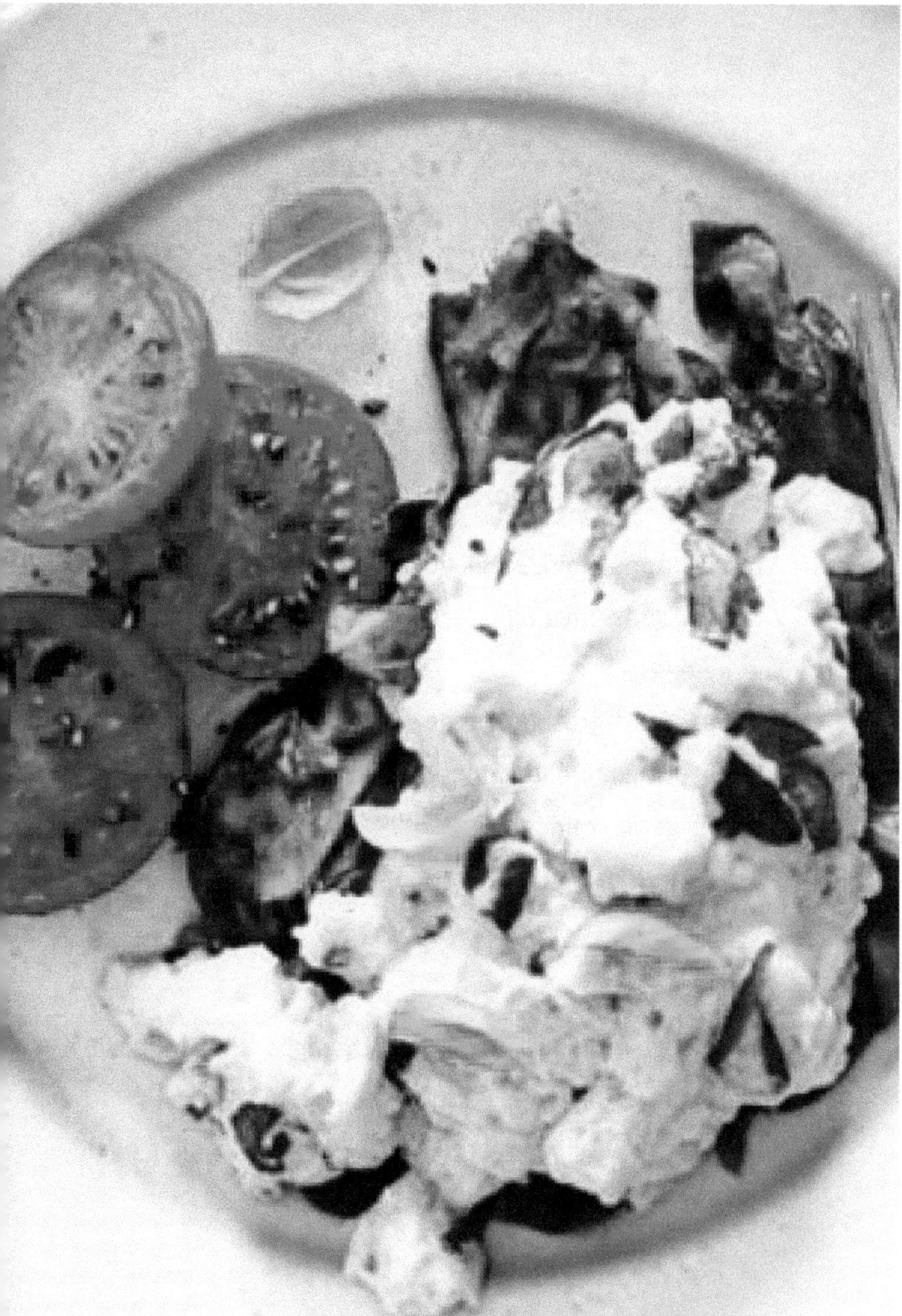

Scrambled Basil Eggs

Servings: 4

Preparation Time: 10 minutes

Per Serving: calories: 243 | fat: 19.7g | protein: 15.6g | carbs: 3.4g | fiber: 0.1g | sodium: 568mg

Ingredients:

- 2 tablespoons plain Greek yogurt
- 2 tablespoons olive oil
- 8 large eggs
- 4 tablespoons grated Gruyère cheese
- 4 tablespoons finely chopped fresh basil
- 4 cloves garlic, minced
- Sea salt and freshly ground pepper, to taste

Procedure:

1. Take a large bowl, beat together the eggs, cheese, basil, and yogurt with a whisk until just combined.
2. Then heat the oil in a large, heavy nonstick skillet over medium-low heat.

3. Now add the garlic and cook until golden, about 1 minute.
4. Pour the egg mixture into the skillet over the garlic. Work the eggs continuously and cook until fluffy and soft.
5. Season with sea salt and freshly ground pepper to taste.
6. Divide between 2 plates and serve immediately.

Apple & Kale Smoothie

Servings: 4

Preparation Time: 5 minutes

Per Serving: calories: 177 | fat: 6.8g | protein: 8.2g | carbs: 22.0g | fiber: 4.1g | sodium: 112mg

Ingredients:

- 1 avocado, diced
- 6 ice cubes
- 4 cups shredded kale
- 1/2 cup 2 percent plain Greek yogurt
- 1 Granny Smith apple, unpeeled, cored and chopped
- 2 cups unsweetened almond milk

Procedure:

1. First, put all ingredients in a blender and blend until smooth and thick.
2. Then pour into two glasses and serve immediately.

Pine Nuts Tahini Toast

Servings: 4

Preparation Time: 10 minutes

Per Serving: calories 142, fat 7.6, fiber 2.7, carbs 13.7, protein 5.8

Ingredients:

- 4 whole wheat bread slices, toasted
- 2 teaspoons water
- Juice of 1 lemon
- 4 teaspoons pine nuts
- A pinch of black pepper
- 2 tablespoons tahini paste
- 4 teaspoons feta cheese, crumbled

Procedure:

1. Take a bowl, mix the tahini with the water and the lemon juice, whisk really well and spread over the toasted bread slices.
2. Top each serving with the remaining ingredients and serve for breakfast.

Dried Cranberries Cinnamon Oatmeal

Servings: 4

Preparation Time: 12 minutes

Per Serving: calories: 107 | fat: 2.1g | protein: 3.2g | carbs: 18.2g | fiber: 4.1g | sodium: 122mg

Ingredients:

- 1 cup dried cranberries
- 2 teaspoons ground cinnamon
- 2 cups almond milk
- 2 cups water
- Pinch sea salt
- 2 cups old-fashioned oats

Procedure:

1. Take a medium saucepan over high heat, bring the almond milk, water, and salt to a boil.
2. Then stir in the oats, cranberries, and cinnamon. Reduce the heat to medium and cook for 5 minutes, stirring occasionally.
3. Now remove the oatmeal from the heat. Cover and let it stand for 3 minutes. Stir before serving.

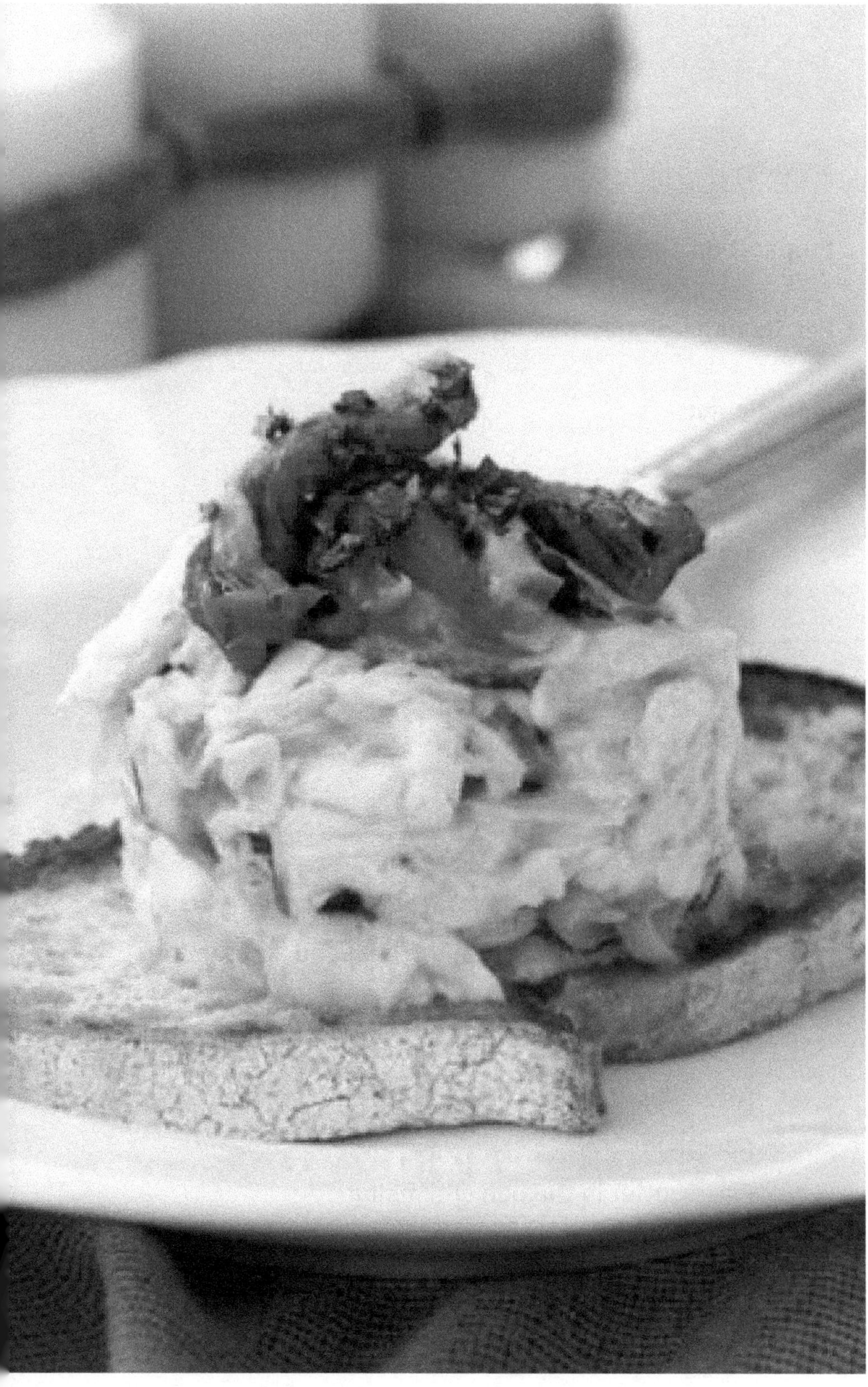

Yummy Chili Scramble

Servings: 8

Preparation Time: 15 minutes

Per Serving: calories 105, fat 7.4, fiber 1.1, carbs 4, protein 6.4

Ingredients:

- 2 tablespoons butter
- 2 cups water, for cooking
- 6 tomatoes
- 8 eggs
- 1/2 teaspoon of sea salt
- 1 chili pepper, chopped

Procedure:

1. First, pour water in the saucepan and bring it to a boil.
2. Then remove water from the heat and add tomatoes.
3. Now let the tomatoes stay in the hot water for 2-3 minutes.
4. After this, remove the tomatoes from the water and peel them.
5. Place butter in the pan and melt it.

6. Add chopped chili pepper and fry it for 3 minutes over medium heat.
7. Then chop the peeled tomatoes and add them into the chili peppers.
8. Cook the vegetables for 5 minutes over medium heat. Stir them from time to time.
9. After this, add sea salt and crack, then eggs.
10. Stir (scramble) the eggs well with the help of the fork and cook them for 3 minutes over medium heat.

Salmon Paprika Toast

Servings: 4

Preparation Time: 3 minutes

Per Serving: calories 202, fat 4.7, fiber 5.1, carbs 31.5, protein 12.7

Ingredients:

- 1 teaspoon paprika
- 8 lettuce leaves
- 2 cucumber, sliced
- 4 teaspoons cream cheese
- 2 teaspoons fresh dill, chopped
- 1 teaspoon lemon juice
- 8 whole grain bread slices
- 4 oz smoked salmon, sliced

Procedure:

1. First, toast the bread in the toaster (1-2 minutes totally).
2. Take the bowl, mix up together fresh dill, cream cheese, lemon juice, and paprika.

3. Then spread the toasts with the cream cheese mixture.
4. Now slice the smoked salmon and place it on 2 bread slices.
5. Add sliced cucumber and lettuce leaves.
6. Top the lettuce with remaining bread toasts and pin with the toothpick.

LUNCH

Beef Chili Jalapeno

Servings: 8

Preparation Time: 50 minutes

Per Serving: Calories 217 Fat 6.1 g Carbohydrates 6.2 g Sugar 2.7 g Protein 33.4 g Cholesterol 92 mg

Ingredients:

- 4 tomatillos, chopped
- 1/2 onion, chopped
- 1 lb ground beef
- 1 tsp garlic powder
- 1 jalapeno pepper, chopped
- 1 lb ground pork
- 5 oz tomato paste
- Pepper
- 1 tbsp ground cumin
- 1 tbsp chili powder
- Salt

Procedure:

1. First, add oil into the instant pot and set the pot on sauté mode.
2. Then add beef and pork and cook until brown.
3. Add remaining ingredients and stir well.
4. Now seal the pot with a lid and cook on high for 35 minutes.
5. Once done, allow to release pressure naturally. Remove lid.
6. Stir well and serve.

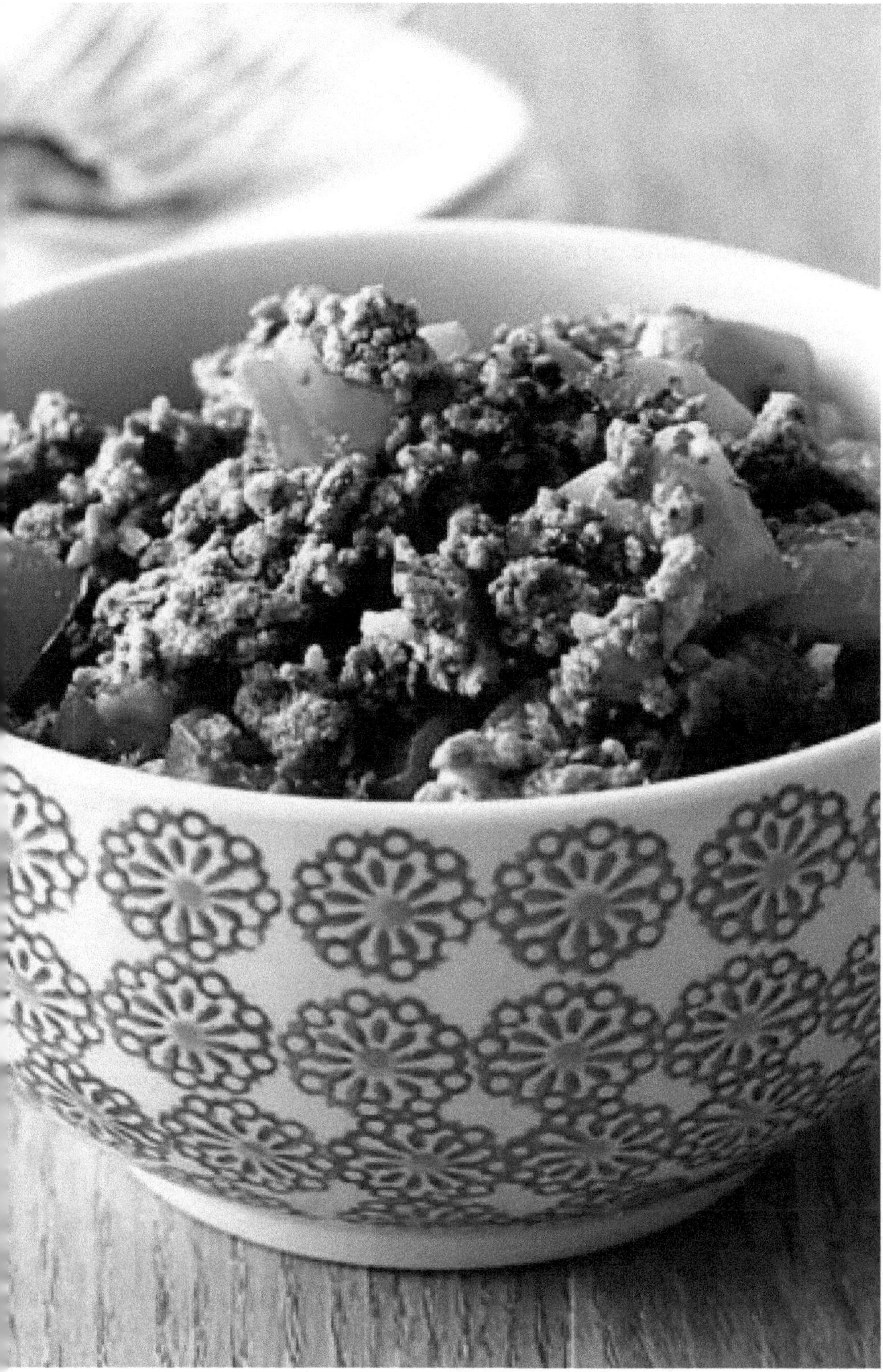

Beef with Tomatoes

Servings: 8

Preparation Time: 50 minutes

Per Serving: Calories 511 Fat 21.6 g Carbohydrates 5.6 g Sugar 2.5 g Protein 70.4 g Cholesterol 203 mg

Ingredients:

- 4 tbsps olive oil
- 2 onions, chopped
- 2 cups beef stock
- 4 lbs beef roast, sliced
- 2 tbsps chives, chopped
- 2 tbsps oregano, chopped
- 2 cups tomatoes, chopped
- Pepper
- Salt
- 2 tsps garlic, minced
- 1 tsp chili powder

Procedure:

1. First, add oil into the instant pot and set the pot on sauté mode.
2. Then add garlic, onion, and chili powder and sauté for 5 minutes.
3. Add meat and cook for 5 minutes.
4. Now add remaining ingredients and stir well.
5. Seal pot with lid and cook on high for 30 minutes.
6. Once done, allow to release pressure naturally for 10 minutes, then release remaining using quick release. Remove lid.
7. Stir well and serve.

Midday Beef Goulash

Servings: 4

Preparation Time: 40 minutes

Per Serving: Calories 389 Fat 15.8 g Carbohydrates 19.3 g Sugar 10.7 g Protein 43.2 g Cholesterol 101 mg

Ingredients:

- 3 tbsps olive oil
- 4 cups chicken broth
- Pepper
- Salt
- 1 cup sun-dried tomatoes, chopped
- 1/2 zucchini, chopped
- 1 lb beef stew meat, cubed
- 2 tbsps olive oil
- 1 onion, chopped
- 1 cabbage, sliced

Procedure:

1. First, add oil into the instant pot and set the pot on sauté mode.

2. Then add onion and sauté for 3-5 minutes.
3. Add tomatoes and cook for 5 minutes.
4. Add remaining ingredients and stir well.
5. Now seal the pot with a lid and cook on high for 20 minutes.
6. Once done, allow to release pressure naturally for 10 minutes, then release remaining using quick release. Remove lid.

Parmesan Stuffed Zucchini Boats

Servings: 8

Preparation Time: 20 minutes

Per Serving: calories: 139 | fat: 4.0g | protein: 8.0g | carbs: 20.0g | fiber: 5.0g | sodium: 344mg

Ingredients:

- 4 zucchinis
- 1/2 cup shredded Parmesan cheese
- 2 cups canned low-sodium chickpeas, drained and rinsed
- 2 cups no-sugar-added spaghetti sauce

Procedure:

1. First, preheat the oven to 425ºF (220ºC).
2. Take a medium bowl, stir together the chickpeas and spaghetti sauce.
3. Then cut the zucchini in half lengthwise and scrape a spoon gently down the length of each half to remove the seeds.

4. Now fill each zucchini half with the chickpea sauce and top with one-quarter of the Parmesan cheese.
5. Place the zucchini halves on a baking sheet and roast in the oven for 15 minutes.
6. Transfer to a plate. Let rest for 5 minutes before serving.

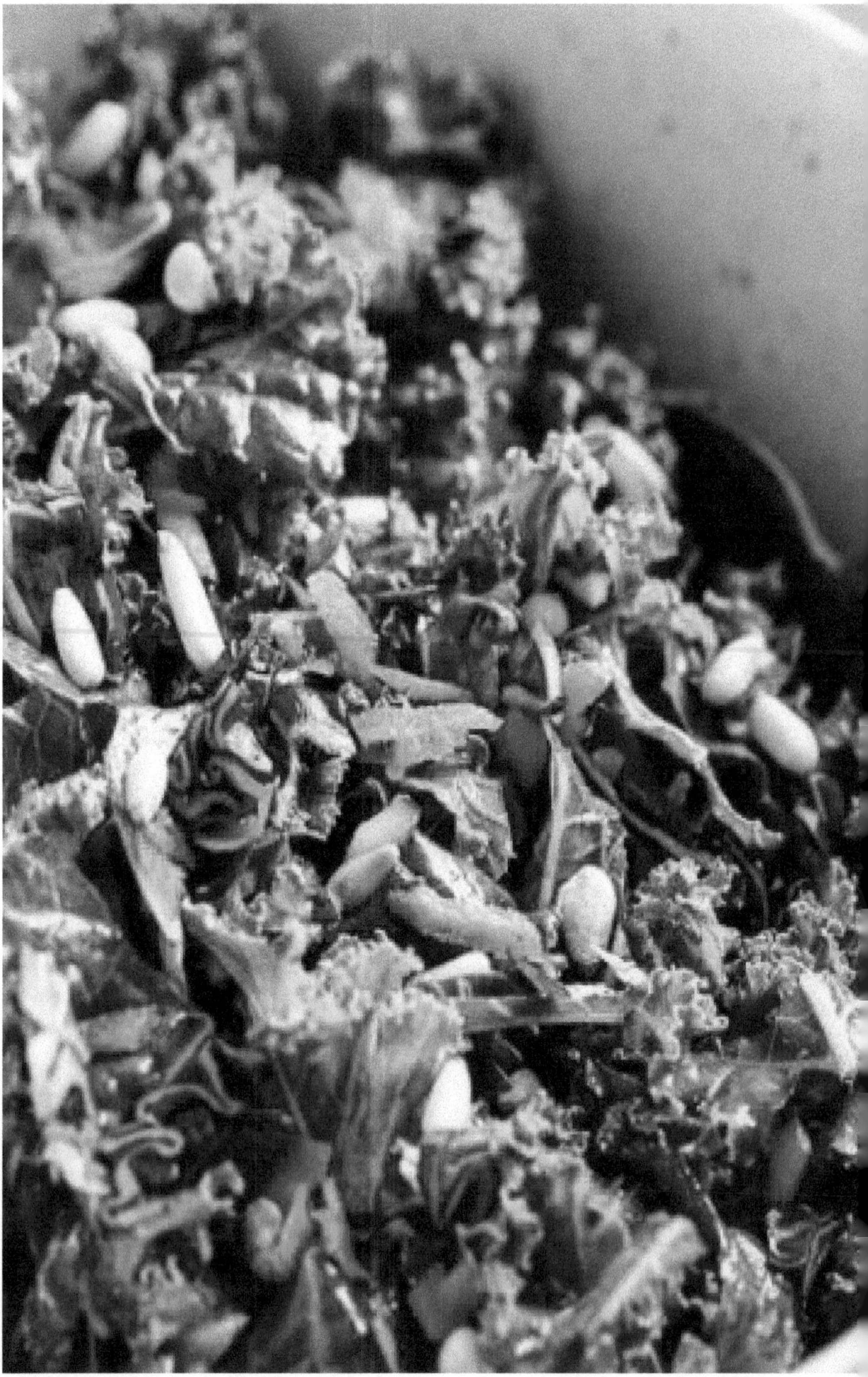

Kale& Cabbage Salad

Servings: 12

Preparation Time: 10 minutes

Per Serving: calories: 199 | fat: 12.0g | protein: 10.0g | carbs: 17.0g | fiber: 5.0g | sodium: 46mg

Ingredients:

- 2 garlic cloves, thinly sliced
- 2 cups toasted peanuts
- 4 bunches baby kale, thinly sliced
- 1 head green savoy cabbage, cored and thinly sliced
- 2 medium red bell peppers, thinly sliced

Dressing:

- 2 teaspoons ground cumin
- 1/2 teaspoon smoked paprika
- Juice of 2 lemons
- 1/2 cup apple cider vinegar

Procedure:

1. Take a large mixing bowl, toss together the kale and cabbage.

Then make the dressing:

2. Whisk together the lemon juice, vinegar, cumin and paprika in a small bowl.
3. Now pour the dressing over the greens and gently massage with your hands.
4. Add the pepper, garlic and peanuts to the mixing bowl. Toss to combine.

Tempting Grilled Romaine Lettuce

Servings: 4

Preparation Time: 10 minutes

Per Serving: calories: 126 | fat: 11.0g | protein: 2.0g | carbs: 7.0g | fiber: 1.0g | sodium: 41mg

Ingredients:

Romaine:

- 2 heads romaine lettuce, halved lengthwise
- 2 tablespoons extra-virgin olive oil

Dressing:

- 1 garlic clove, pressed
- 1 pinch red pepper flakes
- ½ cup unsweetened almond milk
- 1 tablespoon extra-virgin olive oil
- ¼ bunch fresh chives, thinly chopped

Procedure:

1. First, heat a grill pan over medium heat.

2. Then brush each lettuce half with the olive oil.

3. Place the lettuce halves, flat-side down, on the grill.

4. Then grill for 3 to 5 minutes, or until the lettuce slightly wilts and develops light grill marks.

5. Meanwhile, whisk together all the ingredients for the dressing in a small bowl.

6. Now drizzle 2 tablespoons of the dressing over each romaine half and serve.

Mushroom Butter Noodle

Servings: 8

Preparation Time: 20 minutes

Per Serving: calories: 244 | fat: 14.0g | protein: 4.0g | carbs: 22.0g | fiber: 4.0g | sodium: 159mg

Ingredients:

- 2 teaspoons dried thyme
- 1 teaspoon sea salt
- 1/2 cup extra-virgin olive oil
- 2 pounds (900 g) cremini mushrooms, sliced
- 1 red onion, finely chopped
- Pinch of red pepper flakes
- 8 cups butternut noodles
- 8 ounces (220 g) grated Parmesan cheese
- 6 garlic cloves, minced
- 1 cup dry white wine

Procedure:

1. In a large skillet over medium-high heat, heat the olive oil until shimmering.

2. Add the mushrooms, onion, thyme, and salt to the skillet.
3. Cook for about 6 minutes, stirring occasionally, or until the mushrooms start to brown.
4. Add the garlic and sauté for 30 seconds.
5. Stir in the white wine and red pepper flakes.
6. Fold in the noodles.
7. Cook for about 5 minutes, stirring occasionally, or until the noodles are tender.
8. Serve topped with the grated Parmesan.

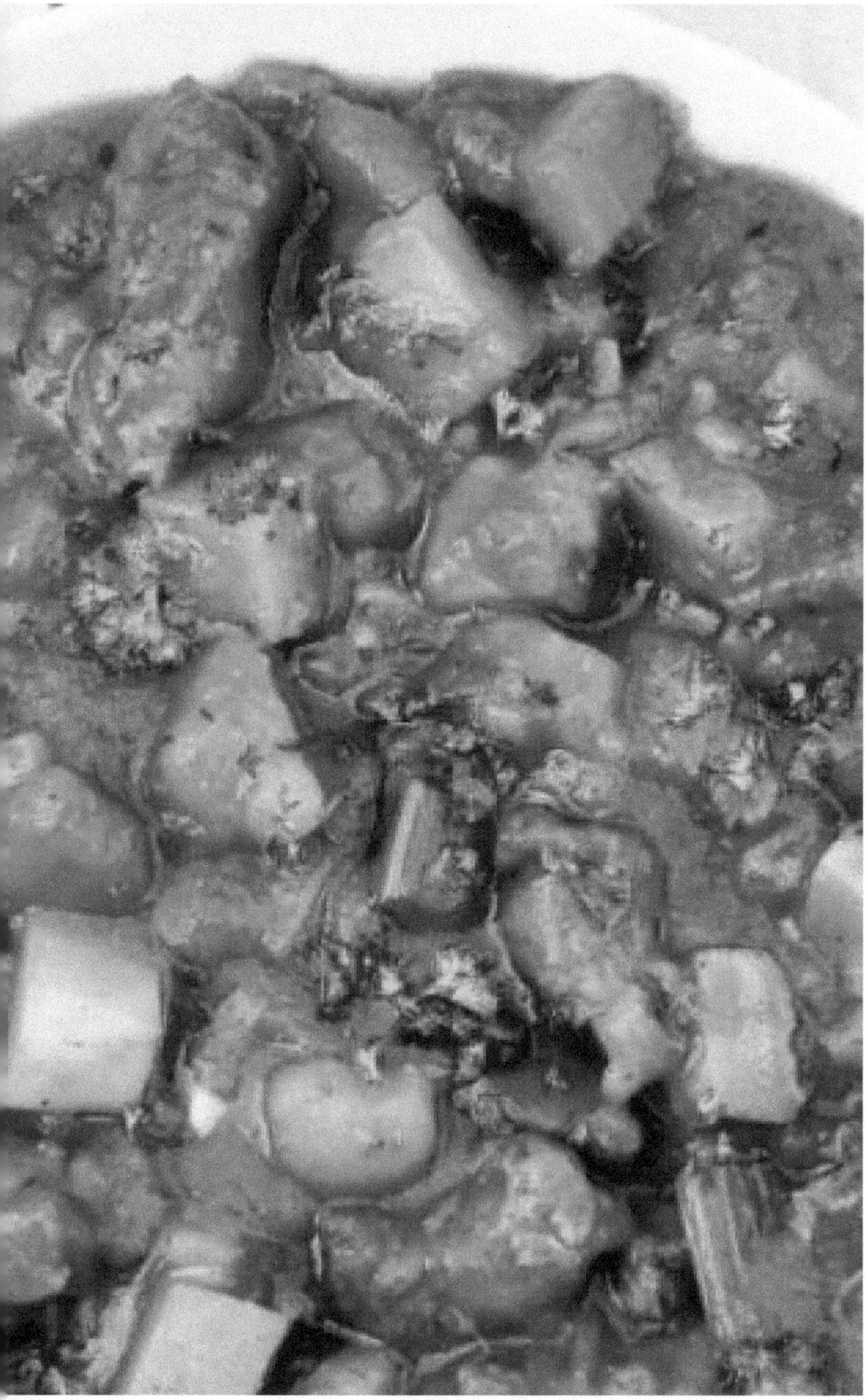

Beans & Sage Pork Stew

Servings: 4

Preparation Time: 4 hours

Per Serving: calories 423, fat 15.4, fiber 9.6, carbs 27.4, protein 43

Ingredients:

- 3 garlic cloves, minced
- 2 teaspoons sage, dried
- 4 ounces canned white beans, drained
- 1 cup beef stock
- 2 pounds pork stew meat, cubed
- 1 sweet onion, chopped
- 1 red bell pepper, chopped
- 2 zucchinis, chopped
- 2 tablespoons olive oil
- 2 tablespoons tomato paste
- 1 tablespoon cilantro, chopped

Procedure:

1. First, heat up a pan with the oil over medium-high heat, add the meat, brown for 10 minutes and transfer to your slow cooker.
2. Then add the rest of the ingredients except the cilantro, put the lid on and cook on High for 4 hours.
3. Divide the stew into bowls, sprinkle the cilantro on top and serve.

Pesto & Broccoli Spaghetti

Servings: 8

Preparation Time: 35 minutes

Per Serving: Calories:284   Fat:10.2g   Protein:10.4g
Carbohydrates:40.2g

Ingredients:

- 8 basil leaves
- 4 tablespoons blanched almonds
- 2 lemons, juiced
- 16 oz. spaghetti
- 2 pounds broccoli, cut into florets
- 4 tablespoons olive oil
- 8 garlic cloves, chopped
- Salt and pepper to taste

Procedure:

1. Firstly, for the pesto, combine the broccoli, oil, garlic, basil, lemon juice and almonds in a blender and pulse until well mixed and smooth.

2. Then cook the spaghetti in a large pot of salty water for 8 minutes or until al dente.
3. Drain well.
4. Mix the warm spaghetti with the broccoli pesto and serve right away.

Stuffed Chicken Chorizo Breast

Servings: 8

Preparation Time: 1 ½ hours

Per Serving: Calories:435   Fat:30.8g   Protein:30.2g
Carbohydrates:4.2g

Ingredients:

- 2 cans diced tomatoes
- 1 cup dry white wine
- 1 cup vegetable stock
- 8 chicken breasts
- 4 chorizo links, diced
- 8 oz. mozzarella, shredded
- 6 tablespoons olive oil
- 2 shallots, chopped
- 4 garlic cloves, minced
- Salt and pepper to taste

Procedure:

1. Mix the chorizo and mozzarella in a bowl.

2. Cut a small pocket into each chicken breast and stuff it with the chorizo.
3. Season the chicken with salt and pepper.
4. Heat the oil in a skillet and add the chicken.
5. Cook on each side for 5 minutes or until golden brown.
6. Add the shallot, garlic and tomatoes, as well as wine, stock, salt and pepper.
7. Cook on low heat for 40 minutes.
8. Serve the chicken and the sauce warm.

Almond, Grapes & Cucumber Soup

Servings: 4

Preparation Time: 10 minutes

Per Serving: calories 200, fat 5.4, fiber 2.4, carbs 7.6, protein 3.3

Ingredients:

- 3 tablespoons olive oil
- Salt and white pepper to the taste
- 1 teaspoon lemon juice
- ¼ cup almonds, chopped and toasted
- 3 cucumbers, peeled and chopped
- 3 garlic cloves, minced
- 6 scallions, sliced
- ¼ cup white wine vinegar
- ½ cup green grapes, halved
- ½ cup warm water

Procedure:

1. Take your blender, combine the almonds with the cucumbers and the rest of the ingredients except the

grapes and lemon juice, pulse well and divide into bowls.

2. Top each serving with the lemon juice and grapes and serve cold.

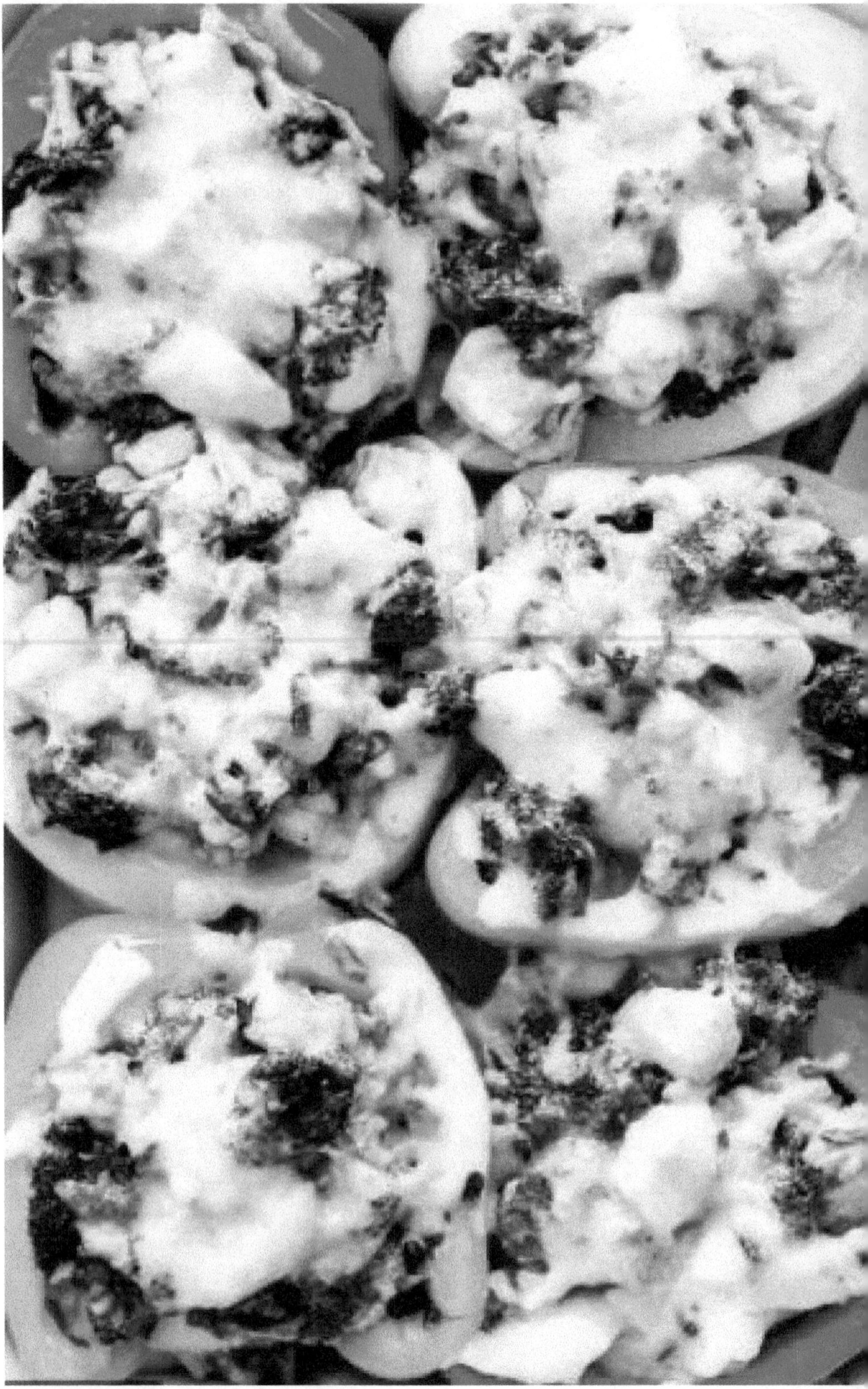

Chicken Stuffed Peppers

Servings: 12

Preparation Time: 10 minutes

Per Serving: calories 266, fat 12.2, fiber 4.5, carbs 15.7, protein 3.7

Ingredients:

- 2 cucumbers, sliced
- 6 red bell peppers, halved and deseeded
- 2 pints cherry tomatoes, quartered
- 2 cups Greek yogurt
- 4 tablespoons mustard
- 4 tablespoons balsamic vinegar
- 2 bunches scallions, sliced
- 1/2 cup parsley, chopped
- Salt and black pepper to the taste
- 2 pounds rotisserie chicken meat, cubed
- 8 celery stalks, chopped

Procedure:

1. Take a bowl, mix the chicken with the celery and the rest of the ingredients except the bell peppers and toss well.
2. Stuff the peppers halves with the chicken mix and serve for lunch.

DINNER

Quick Shrimp

Servings: 12

Preparation Time: 10 minutes

Per Serving: Calories 165 Fat 2.4 g Carbohydrates 2.2 g Sugar 0.1 g Protein 30.6 g Cholesterol 279 mg

Ingredients:

- 3 1/2 lbs shrimp, frozen and deveined
- 1 cup fish stock
- 1 cup apple cider vinegar
- Pepper
- Salt

Procedure:

1. First, add all ingredients into the inner pot of instant pot and stir well.
2. Then seal the pot with a lid and cook on high for 1 minute.
3. Once done, release pressure using quick release.
4. Remove lid.
5. Stir and serve.

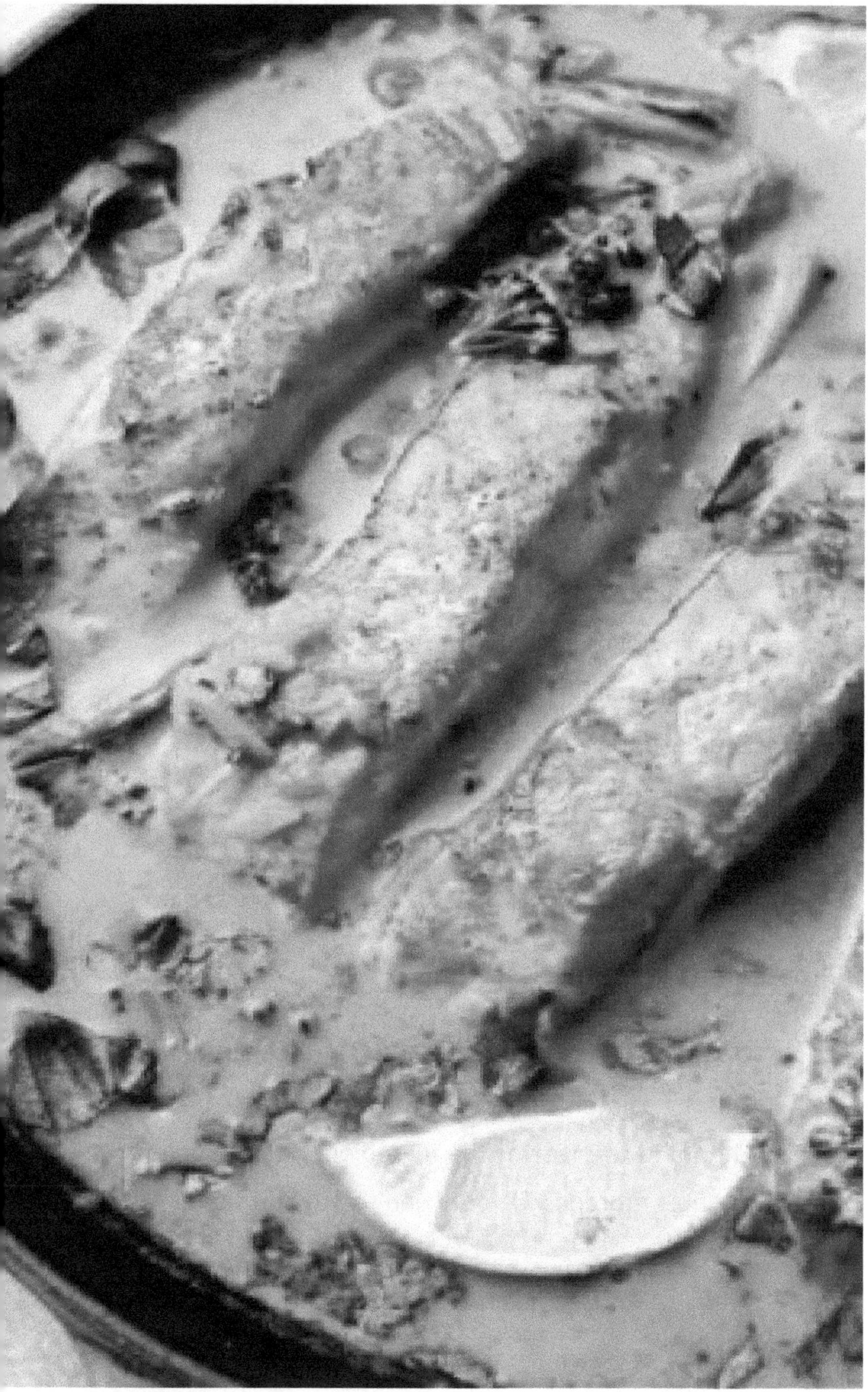

Creamy Salmon Curry

Servings: 4

Preparation Time: 30 minutes

Per Serving: Calories 284, fat 14.1, fiber 8.5, carbs 26.7, protein 31.4

Ingredients:

- 2 cups Greek yogurt
- 4 teaspoons curry powder
- 2 garlic cloves, minced
- 1 teaspoon mint, chopped
- 2 tablespoons basil, chopped
- Sea salt and black pepper to the taste
- 4 salmon fillets, boneless and cubed
- 2 tablespoons olive oil

Procedure:

1. First, heat up a pan with the oil over medium-high heat, add the salmon and cook for 3 minutes.
2. Then add the rest of the ingredients, toss, cook for 15 minutes more, divide between plates and serve.

Veggie Mix & Smoked Salmon

Servings: 8

Preparation Time: 30 minutes

Per Serving: Calories 301, fat 5.9, fiber 11.9, carbs 26.4, protein 22.4

Ingredients:

- 8 salmon fillets, skinless and boneless
- 4 tablespoons chives, chopped
- 6 red onions, cut into wedges
- 1 1/2 cups green olives, pitted and halved
- Salt and black pepper to the taste
- 6 tablespoons olive oil
- 6 red bell peppers, roughly chopped
- 1 teaspoon smoked paprika

Procedure:

1. Take a roasting pan, combine the salmon with the onions and the rest of the ingredients, introduce in the oven and bake at 390 degrees F for 20 minutes.
2. Divide the mix between plates and serve.

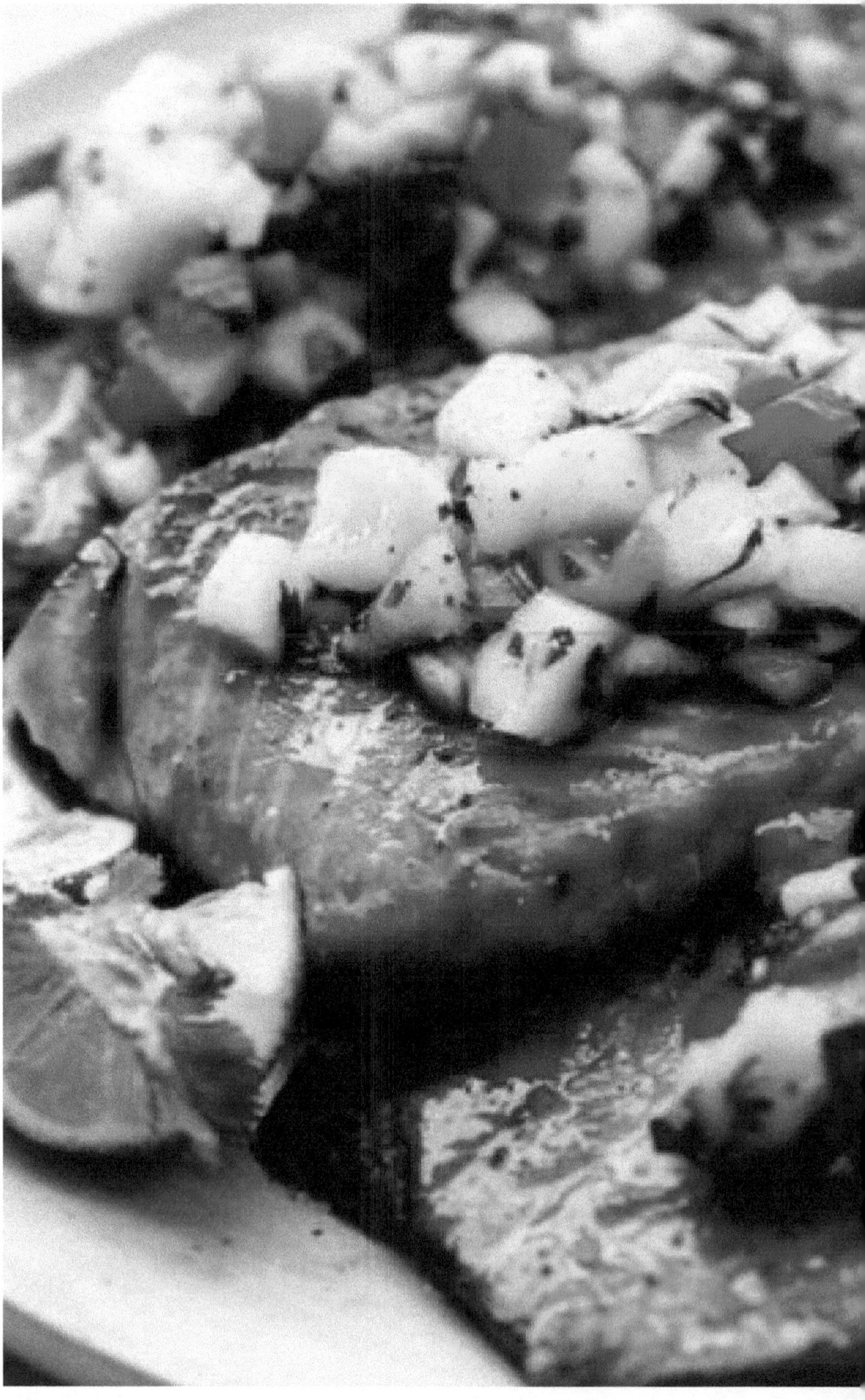

Mango & Salmon Mix

Servings: 4

Preparation Time: 35 minutes

Per Serving: Calories 251, fat 15.9, fiber 5.9, carbs 26.4, protein 12.4

Ingredients:

- 2 small piece gingers, grated
- Juice of 1 lime
- 2 tablespoons cilantro, chopped
- 4 salmon fillets, skinless and boneless
- 4 mangos, peeled and cubed
- 2 red chili, chopped
- Salt and pepper to the taste
- 4 tablespoons olive oil
- 4 garlic cloves, minced

Procedure:

1. Take a roasting pan, combine the salmon with the oil, garlic and the rest of the ingredients except the

cilantro, toss, introduce in the oven at 350 degrees F and bake for 25 minutes.

2. Divide everything between plates and serve with the cilantro sprinkled on top.

Tempting Honey Almond Chicken Tenders

Servings: 4

Preparation Time: 30 minutes

Per Serving: Calories: 263 Protein: 31 Grams Fat: 12 Grams Carbs: 9 Grams.

Ingredients:

- 1 Tablespoon Dijon Mustard.
- 1 Tablespoon Honey, Raw.
- Sea Salt & Black Pepper to Taste.
- 1 Lb. Chicken Breast Tenders, Boneless & Skinless.
- 1 Cup Almonds.

Procedure:

1. First, start by heating your oven to 425, and then get out a baking sheet.
2. Then line it with parchment paper, and then put a cooking rack on it.
3. Spray your cooling rack down with nonstick cooking spray.

4. Now get out a bowl and combine your mustard and honey.
5. Season with salt and pepper, and then add in your chicken.
6. After that, make sure it's well coated and place it to the side.
7. Use a knife and chop your almonds.
8. You can also use a food processor.
9. You want them to roughly be the same size as sunflower seeds.
10. Press your chicken into the almonds, and then lay it on your cooking rack.
11. Bake for fifteen to twenty minutes.
12. Your chicken should be cooked all the way through.

Simple Special Chops

Servings: 2

Preparation Time: 12 minutes

Per Serving: Calories: 255 Fat: 13.9g Fiber: 0.2g Carbs: 5g Protein: 14.6g.

Ingredients:

- Thyme, ¼ Teaspoon.
- Salt And Pepper As Needed.
- Extra Virgin Olive Oil, 1 Tablespoon.
- Greek Yogurt, 2 Tablespoons.
- 2 Lamb Chops.
- Minced Shallots 2 Tablespoons.
- Balsamic Vinegar, 2 Tablespoons.
- Chicken Broth, 2 Tablespoons.
- Basil, ¼ Teaspoon.
- Rosemary, 1 Teaspoon.

Procedure:

1. First, take a mixing bowl and mix all herbs and yogurt with seasoning.

2. Then rub this mixture into the chops completely. Leave them for a few minutes.

3. Now heat a skillet over medium heat and cook both sides of the chops well.

4. When tender, brown the shallots on the skillet and add the vinegar and broth.

5. Then top the chops with the warm sauce of broth and serve on a platter.

Beef Sushi

Servings: 4

Preparation Time: 35 minutes

Per Serving: Calories: 207 Fat: 13.4g Fiber: 1.6g Carbs: 5.5g Protein: 16.4g.

Ingredients:

- Stock, 1/2 Cup.
- Soy Sauce, 2 Teaspoons.
- Beef, 1 Pound, Sliced.
- Extra Virgin Olive Oil, 2 Teaspoons.
- Onion, 1/2 Cup, Diced.
- Spinach, Fresh, 4 Ounces.
- Celery, 4 Tablespoons, Diced.
- Mushrooms, 4 Ounces, Chopped.

Procedure:

1. First, take a wok and the heating oil. Add beef, and stir.
2. Then mix the sauce and toss with the veggies and mushrooms when beef is brown.
3. Now cook well, and then fold in the spinach.
4. Serve after a couple of minutes.

Lemony Grilled Chicken

Servings: 12

Preparation Time: 25 minutes

Per Serving: Calories: 216kcal. Carbohydrates: 2g Protein: 24g. Fat: 12g. Saturated Fat: 2g. Cholesterol: 72mg.

Ingredients:

- 1 Teaspoon Salt.
- 1/2 Teaspoon Pepper.
- Parsley or Cilantro for Serving.
- Lemon Wedges for Serving
- 1/2 Cup Lemon Juice plus the Zest for the Lemons.
- 4 Teaspoons Oregano.
- 8 Garlic Cloves Pressed.
- 12 Ounces Boneless Skinless Chicken Breasts.
- 1/2 Cup Olive Oil.

   Procedure:

1. Pat chicken dry and pound chicken if some parts are too thick.
2. Combine the olive oil, lemon juice, oregano, garlic, salt, and pepper in a bowl or resealable freezer bag.

3. Add chicken and toss well to combine. Marinate for at least 30 minutes.
4. Preheat grill or grill pan to medium-high heat. Place chicken on the grill for 5-7 minutes.
5. Use tongs to flip over and cook until juices run dry, approximately 5-7 more minutes.
6. Discard extra marinade.
7. Remove chicken from the grill.
8. Sprinkle with parsley and serve with lemon wedges and vegetables, if desired.

Yummy Mushroom Pilaf

Servings: 8

Preparation Time: 50 minutes

Per Serving: Calories:265 Fat:8.9g Protein:7.6g Carbohydrates:41.2g

Ingredients:

- 2 thyme sprigs
- 2 bay leafs
- Salt and pepper to taste
- 2 pounds button mushrooms
- 2 cups brown rice
- 4 tablespoons olive oil
- 2 shallots, chopped
- 4 garlic cloves, minced
- 4 cups chicken stock

Procedure:

1. First, heat the oil in a skillet and stir in the shallot and garlic. Cook for 2 minutes until softened and fragrant.

2. Then add the mushrooms and rice and cook for 5 minutes.
3. Now add the stock, bay leaf and thyme, as well as salt and pepper and continue cooking for 20 more minutes on low heat.

Cheese Artichoke Mix

Servings: 6

Preparation Time: 45 minutes

Per Serving: calories 272, fat 17.3, fiber 4.3, carbs 20.2, protein 11.8

Ingredients:

- 1 cup spinach, chopped
- ½ teaspoon salt
- 3 eggs, beaten
- 1 teaspoon canola oil
- ½ cup cottage cheese
- 1 teaspoon ground black pepper
- 3 tablespoons fresh dill, chopped
- 4 sheets matzo
- ½ cup artichoke hearts, canned
- 1 cup cream cheese

Procedure:

1. Take the bowl combine together cream cheese, spinach, salt, ground black pepper, dill, and cottage cheese.
2. Then pour canola oil in the skillet, add artichoke hearts and roast them for 2-3 minutes over medium heat.
3. Now stir them from time to time.
4. Then add roasted artichoke hearts in the cheese mixture.
5. Add eggs and stir until homogenous.
6. Place one sheet of matzo in the casserole mold.
7. Then spread it with cheese mixture generously.
8. Cover the cheese layer with the second sheet of matzo.
9. Repeat the steps till you use all ingredients.
10. Then preheat the oven to 360F.
11. Bake matzo mina for 40 minutes.
12. Cut the cooked meal into the servings.

Shallots Caramelized Steaks

Servings: 12

Preparation Time: 45 minutes

Per Serving: Calories:258 Fat:16.3g Protein:23.5g Carbohydrates:2.1g

Ingredients:

- 8 tablespoons olive oil
- 1/2 cup dry white wine
- 12 flank steaks
- Salt and pepper to taste
- 2 teaspoons dried oregano
- 2 teaspoons dried basil
- 12 shallots, sliced

Procedure:

1. Firstly, season the steaks with salt, pepper, oregano and basil.
2. Then heat a grill pan over medium flame and place the steaks on the grill.
3. Cook on each side for 6-7 minutes.

4. Heat the oil in a skillet and stir in the shallots. Cook for 15 minutes, stirring often, until the shallots are caramelized.
5. Add the wine and cook for another 5 minutes.

Braised Pear Pork

Servings: 10

Preparation Time: 2 ½ hours

Per Serving: Calories:455   Fat:29.3g   Protein:32.1g
Carbohydrates:14.9g

Ingredients:

- 2 shallots, sliced
- 4 garlic cloves, minced
- 1 bay leaf
- 3 pounds pork shoulder
- 4 pears, peeled and sliced
- ½ cup apple cider
- Salt and pepper to taste
- 1 thyme sprig

Procedure:

1. First, season the pork with salt and pepper.
2. Then combine the pears, shallots, garlic, bay leaf, thyme and apple cider in a deep dish baking pan.

3. Now place the pork over the pears, then cover the pan with aluminum foil.
4. Cook in the preheated oven at 330F for 2 hours.

Baked Yogurt Eggplant

Servings: 8

Preparation Time: 45 minutes

Per Serving: Calories:113 Fat:1.6g Protein:8.1g Carbohydrates:19.4g

Ingredients:

- 1 teaspoon dried basil
- 2 tablespoons lemon juice
- Salt and pepper to taste
- 2 eggplants
- 4 garlic cloves, minced
- 1 cup Greek yogurt
- 2 tablespoons chopped parsley

Procedure:

1. First, cut the eggplants in half and score the halves with sharp knives.
2. Then season the eggplants with salt and pepper, as well as the basil, then drizzle with lemon juice and place the eggplant halves on a baking tray.

3. Now spread the garlic over the eggplants and bake in the preheated oven at 350F for 20 minutes.
4. When done, place the eggplants on serving plates and top with yogurt and parsley.

SNACKS

Greek Salad Wraps

Servings: 4

Preparation Time: 15 minutes

Per Serving: calories: 225 | fat: 12.0g | protein: 12.0g | carbs: 18.0g | fiber: 4.0g | sodium: 349mg

Ingredients:

- ½ cup finely chopped fresh mint
- ¼ cup diced red onion
- 1 (2.25-ounce / 64-g) can sliced black olives, drained
- 2 tablespoons extra-virgin olive oil
- 1½ cups seedless cucumber, peeled and chopped
- 1 tablespoon red wine vinegar
- ¼ teaspoon kosher salt
- ¼ teaspoon freshly ground black pepper
- ½ cup crumbled goat cheese
- 4 whole-wheat flatbread wraps or soft whole-wheat tortillas
- 1 cup chopped tomato

Procedure:

1. In a large bowl, stir together the cucumber, tomato, mint, onion and olives.
2. In a small bowl, whisk together the oil, vinegar, salt, and pepper.
3. Spread the dressing over the salad. Toss gently to combine.
4. On a clean work surface, lay the wraps.
5. Divide the goat cheese evenly among the wraps.
6. Scoop a quarter of the salad filling down the center of each wrap.
7. Fold up each wrap: Start by folding up the bottom, then fold one side over and fold the other side over the top.
8. Repeat with the remaining wraps.

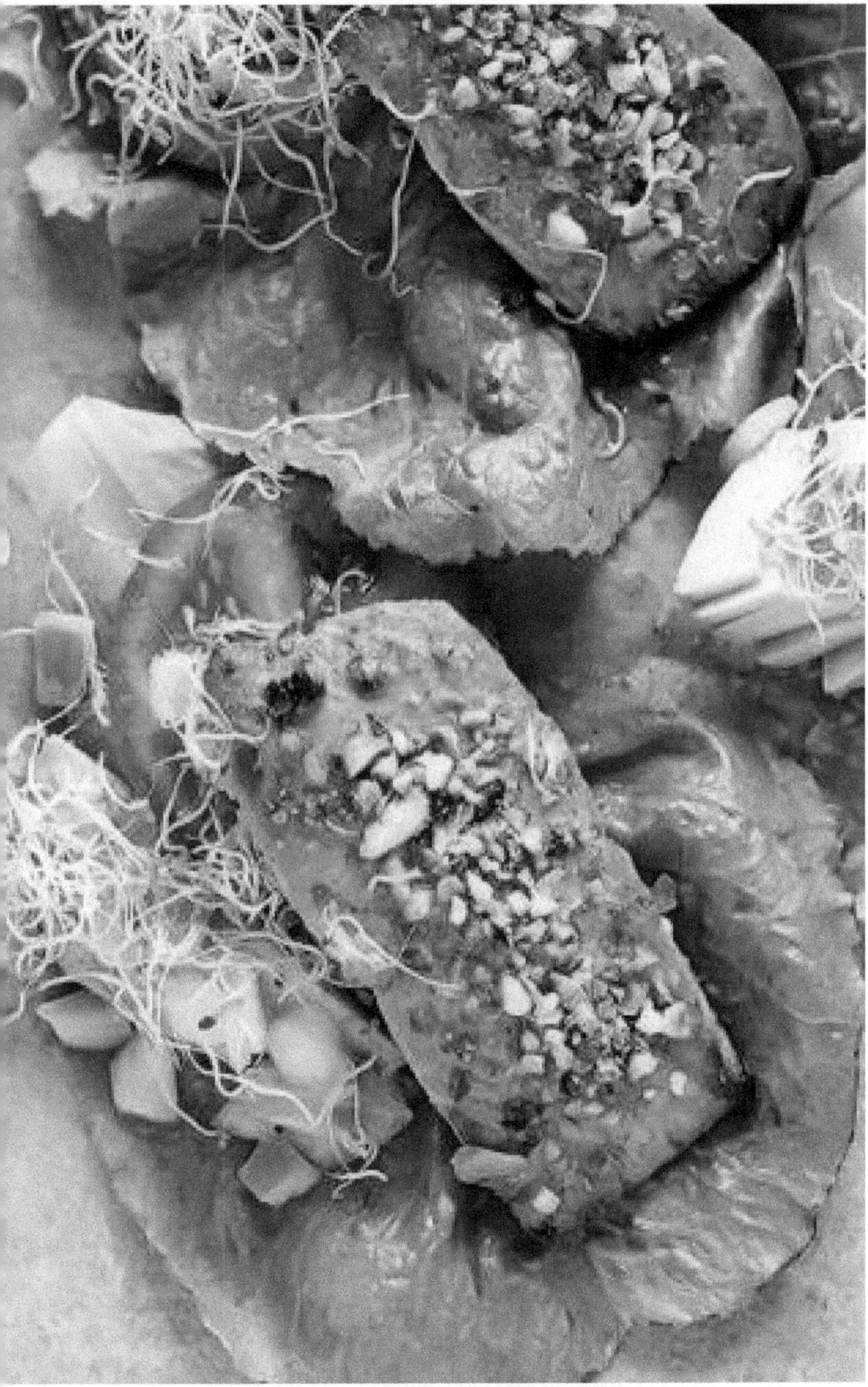

Heart Salmon Salad Wraps

Servings: 6

Preparation Time: 10 minutes

Per Serving: calories: 194 | fat: 8.0g | protein: 18.0g | carbs: 13.0g | fiber: 3.0g | sodium: 536mg

Ingredients:

- 1 pound (454 g) salmon fillets, cooked and flaked
- 1 tablespoon aged balsamic vinegar
- ½ cup diced celery
- 3 tablespoons diced red onion
- 3 tablespoons chopped fresh dill
- 2 tablespoons capers
- 1½ tablespoons extra-virgin olive oil
- ¼ teaspoon kosher or sea salt
- ½ teaspoon freshly ground black pepper
- 4 whole-wheat flatbread wraps or soft whole-wheat tortillas
- ½ cup diced carrots

Procedure:

1. Take a large bowl, stir together all the ingredients, except for the wraps.
2. On a clean work surface, lay the wraps. Divide the salmon mixture evenly among the wraps.
3. Fold up the bottom of the wraps, then roll up the wrap.

Feta, Arugula. & Watermelon Salad

Servings: 4

Preparation Time: 10 minutes

Per Serving: calories: 157 | fat: 6.9g | protein: 6.1g | carbs: 22.0g | fiber: 1.1g | sodium: 328mg

Ingredients:

- 4 ounces (110 g) feta cheese, crumbled
- 4 tablespoons balsamic glaze
- 6 cups packed arugula
- 5 cups watermelon, cut into bite-size cubes

Procedure:

1. First, divide the arugula between two plates.
2. Then divide the watermelon cubes between the beds of arugula.
3. Now scatter half of the feta cheese over each salad.
4. Drizzle about 1 tablespoon of the glaze (or more if desired) over each salad. Serve immediately.

Tomato Hummus Soup

Servings: 4

Preparation Time: 20 minutes

Per Serving: calories: 147 | fat: 6.2g | protein: 5.2g | carbs: 20.1g | fiber: 4.1g | sodium: 682mg

Ingredients:

- 4 cups low-sodium chicken stock
- Salt, to taste
- 2 can crushed tomatoes with basil
- 1/2 cup thinly sliced fresh basil leaves, for garnish (optional)
- 2 cups roasted red pepper hummus

Procedure:

1. Combine the canned tomatoes, hummus, and chicken stock in a blender and blend until smooth. Pour the mixture into a saucepan and bring it to a boil.
2. Season with salt to taste.
3. Serve garnished with the fresh basil, if desired.

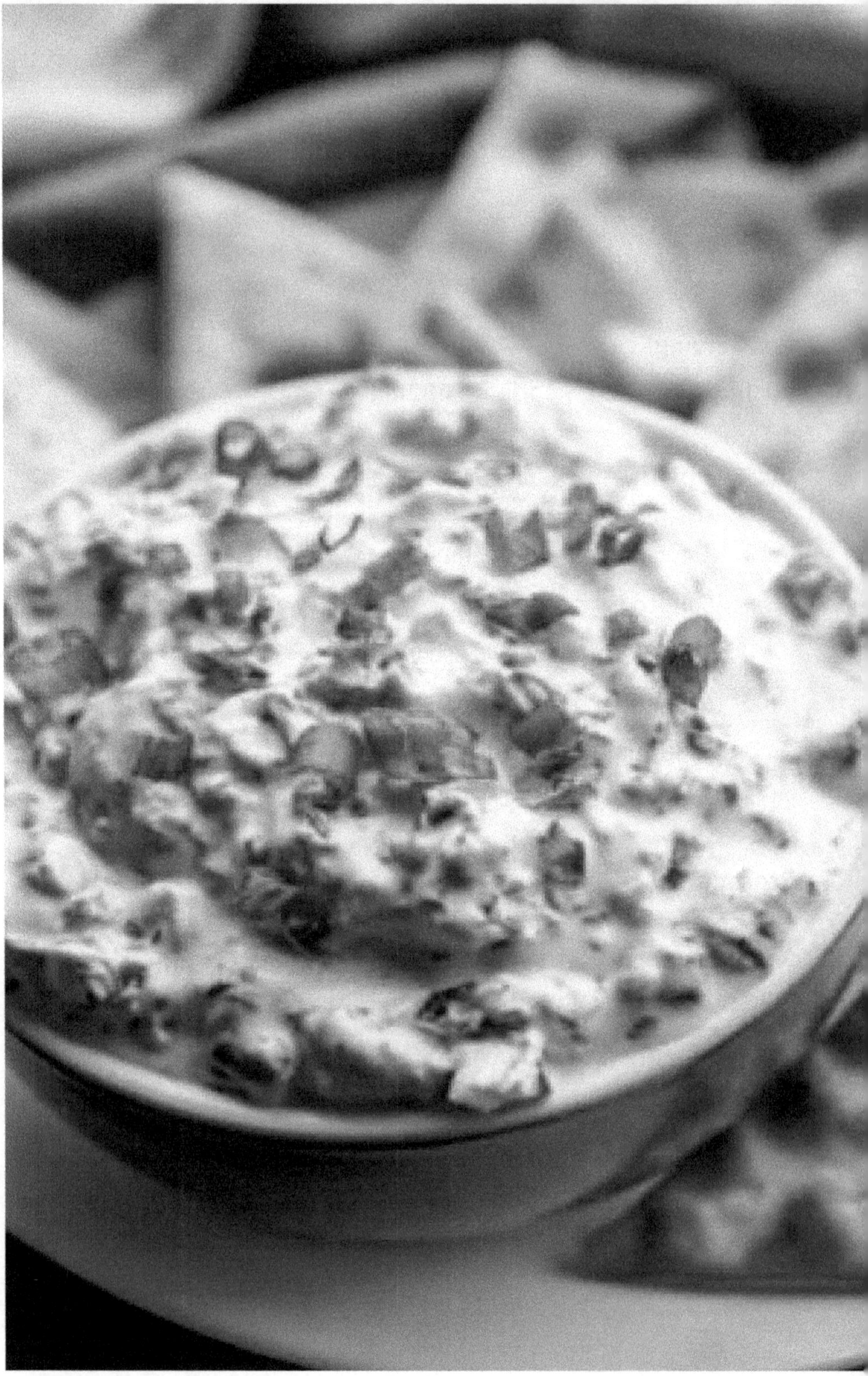

Healthy Scallion Dip

Servings: 16

Preparation Time: 10 minutes

Per Serving: calories 144, fat 7.7, fiber 1.4, carbs 6.3, protein 5.5

Ingredients:

- 2 tablespoons lemon juice
- 3 cups cream cheese, soft
- 4 ounces prosciutto, cooked and crumbled
- 6 tablespoons olive oil
- Salt and black pepper to the taste
- 12 scallions, chopped
- 2 garlic cloves, minced

Procedure:

1. Take a bowl, mix the scallions with the garlic and the rest of the ingredients except the prosciutto and whisk well.
2. Divide into bowls, sprinkle the prosciutto on top and serve as a party dip.

Hearty Layash Roll-Ups

Servings: 3

Preparation Time: 10 minutes

Per Serving: 250 cal, 8 g total fat (0.5 g sat. fat), 0 mg chol., 440 mg sodium, 340 mg pot., 43 total carbs., 40 g fiber, 3 g sugar, 10 g protein, 15% vitamin A, 25% vitamin C, 6% calcium, and 8% iron.

Ingredients:

- 1/2 cup hummus of choice
- 1/2 cup grape tomatoes, halved
- 1 Medium cucumber, sliced
- 1/4 cup black olives, sliced
- Fresh dill, for garnish
- 2 lavash wraps (whole-wheat)
- 1/4 cup roasted red peppers, sliced

Procedure:

1. Lay out the lavash wraps on a clean surface. Evenly spread hummus over each piece.

2. Layer the cucumbers across the wraps, about 1/2-inch from each other, leaving about 2-inch empty space at the bottom of the wrap for rolling purposes.
3. Place the roasted pepper slices around the cucumbers. Sprinkle with black olives and tomatoes.
4. Garnish with freshly chopped dill.
5. Tightly roll each wrap, using the hummus at the end to almost glue the wrap into a roll.
6. Slice each roll into 4 equal pieces.
7. Secure each piece by sticking a toothpick through the center of each roll slice.
8. Lay each on a serving bowl or tray; garnish more with fresh dill.

Eggplant & Chickpea Bowl

Servings: 8

Preparation Time: 10 minutes

Per Serving: calories 263, fat 12, fiber 9.3, carbs 15.4, protein 7.5

Ingredients:

- 2 bunches parsley, chopped
- A pinch of salt and black pepper
- 2 tablespoons balsamic vinegar
- 4 eggplants, cut in half lengthwise and cubed
- 2 tablespoons olive oil
- 56 ounces canned chickpeas, drained and rinsed
- 2 red onions, chopped
- Juice of 2 limes

Procedure:

1. Firstly, spread the eggplant cubes on a baking sheet lined with parchment paper, drizzle half of the oil all over, season with salt and pepper and cook at 425 degrees F for 10 minutes.

2. Then cool the eggplant down, add the rest of the ingredients, toss, divide between appetizer plates and serve.

Beet Vinegar Bites

Servings: 8

Preparation Time: 30 minutes

Per Serving: calories 199, fat 5.4, fiber 3.5, carbs 8.5, protein 3.5

Ingredients:

- 2 cups olive oil
- 4 beets, sliced
- A pinch of sea salt and black pepper
- 2/3 cup balsamic vinegar

Procedure:

1. First, spread the beet slices on a baking sheet lined with parchment paper, add the rest of the ingredients, toss and bake at 350 degrees F for 30 minutes.
2. Serve the beet bites cold as a snack.

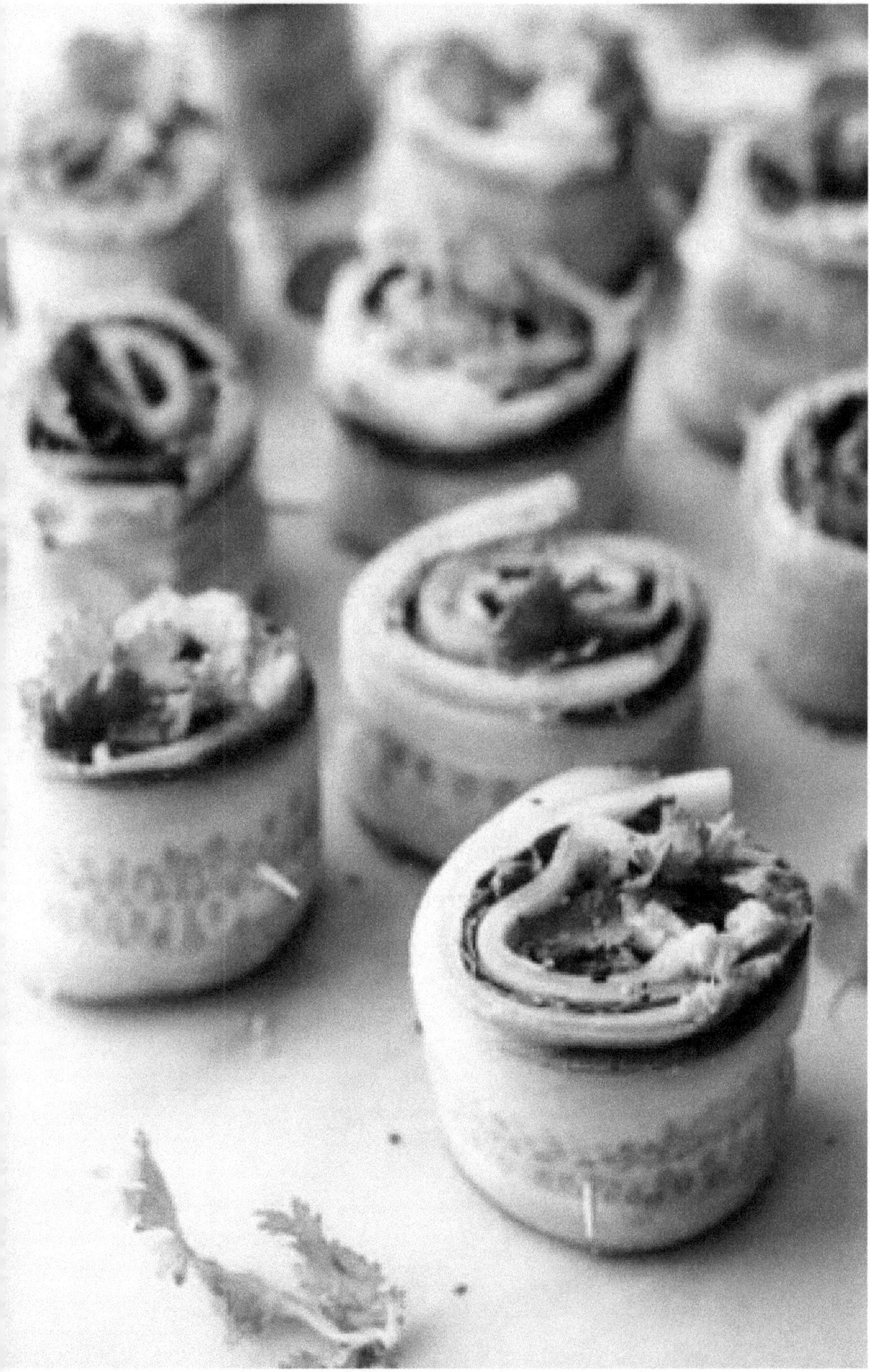

Healthy Cucumber Rolls

Servings: 12

Preparation Time: 20 minutes

Per Serving: calories 200, fat 6, fiber 3.4, carbs 7.6, protein 3.5

Ingredients:

- 2 tablespoons parsley, chopped
- Salt and black pepper to the taste
- 2 big cucumbers, sliced lengthwise
- 2 teaspoons lime juice
- 16 ounces canned tuna, drained and mashed

Procedure:

1. First, arrange cucumber slices on a working surface, divide the rest of the ingredients, and roll.
2. Then arrange all the rolls on a platter and serve as an appetizer.

Easy Roasted Baby Potatoes

Servings: 8

Preparation Time: 20 minutes

Per Serving: Calories 175 Fat 4.5 g Carbohydrates 29.8 g Sugar 0.7 g Protein 6.1 g Cholesterol 2 mg

Ingredients:

- 4 tsps Italian seasoning
- 2 tbsps olive oil
- Pepper
- 4 lbs baby potatoes, clean and cut in half
- 1 cup vegetable stock
- 2 tsps onion powder
- Salt
- 2 tsps paprika
- 1 1/2 tsps garlic powder

Procedure:

1. First, add oil into the inner pot of instant pot and set the pot on sauté mode.

2. Then add potatoes and sauté for 5 minutes. Add remaining ingredients and stir well.
3. Now seal the pot with a lid and cook on high for 5 minutes.
4. Once done, release pressure using quick release. Remove lid.
5. Stir well and serve.

Italian Potatoes

Servings: 12

Preparation Time: 20 minutes

Per Serving: Calories 149 Fat 0.3 g Carbohydrates 41.6 g Sugar 11.4 g Protein 4.5 g Cholesterol 0 mg

Ingredients:

4 lbs baby potatoes, clean and cut in half

1 1/2 cups vegetable broth

12 oz Italian dry dressing mix

Procedure:

1. First, add all ingredients into the inner pot of instant pot and stir well.
2. Then seal the pot with a lid and cook on high for 7 minutes.
3. Once done, allow to release pressure naturally for 3 minutes, then release remaining using quick release. Remove lid.
4. Stir well and serve.

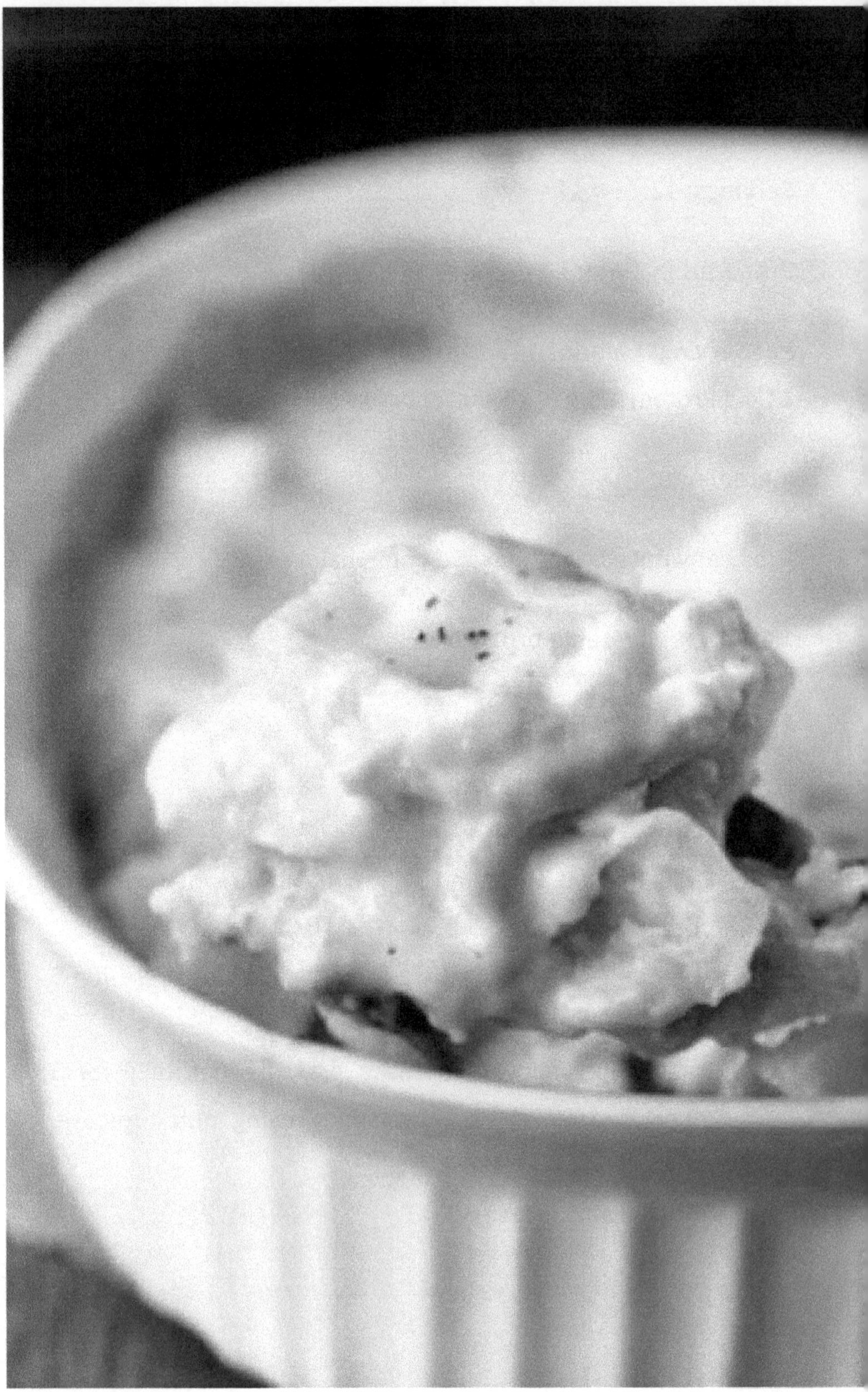

Potato Creamy Spread

Servings: 12

Preparation Time: 25 minutes

Per Serving: Calories 108 Fat 0.3 g Carbohydrates 25.4 g Sugar 2.4 g Protein 2 g Cholesterol 0 mg

Ingredients:

- 1 tsp paprika
- 2 tbsps garlic, minced
- 2 lb sweet potatoes, peeled and chopped
- 1 1/2 tbsps fresh chives, chopped
- 2 cups tomato puree
- Pepper
- Salt

Procedure:

1. First, add all ingredients except chives into the inner pot of instant pot and stir well.
2. Then seal the pot with a lid and cook on high for 15 minutes.

3. Once done, allow to release pressure naturally for 10 minutes, then release remaining using quick release. Remove lid.
4. Now transfer instant pot sweet potato mixture into the food processor and process until smooth.
5. Garnish with chives and serve.

Cucumber Tomato Okra Salsa

Servings: 4

Preparation Time: 25 minutes

Per Serving: Calories 99 Fat 4.2 g Carbohydrates 14.3 g Sugar 6.4 g Protein 2.9 g Cholesterol 0 mg

Ingredients:

- 1 tbsp fresh oregano, chopped
- 1 tbsp fresh basil, chopped
- 1 lb tomatoes, chopped
- 1/4 tsp red pepper flakes
- 1 onion, chopped
- 1 tbsp olive oil
- 1 tbsp garlic, chopped
- 1 1/2 cups okra, chopped
- Pepper
- Salt
- 1/4 cup fresh lemon juice
- 1 cucumber, chopped

Procedure:

1. Add oil into the inner pot of instant pot and set the pot on sauté mode.
2. Add onion, garlic, pepper, and salt and sauté for 3 minutes.
3. Add remaining ingredients except for cucumber and stir well.
4. Seal pot with lid and cook on high for 12 minutes.
5. Once done, allow to release pressure naturally for 10 minutes, then release remaining using quick release. Remove lid.
6. Once the salsa mixture is cool, then add cucumber and mix well.

Lightning Source UK Ltd.
Milton Keynes UK
UKHW020740170521
383851UK00001B/79